D1643596

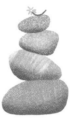

Destination
WELLNESS

Kate Morgan
Illustrations by Wenjia Tang

Hardie Grant

TRAVEL

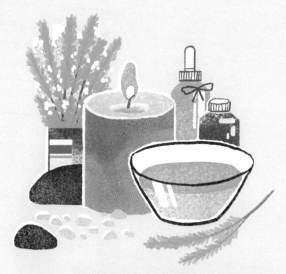

Destination
WELLNESS

Contents

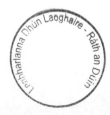

Introduction

It's no secret: the wellness industry is booming. It's hard to go one day without hearing about it in some form or another, from the latest protein powders and plant-based diets to specialised health retreats and digital detoxes. But what does this buzzword 'wellness' mean? The *Oxford English Dictionary* defines it as 'the state of being in good health, especially as an actively pursued goal'. So, despite all the noise, hype and latest gadgets surrounding wellness, what it comes down to is looking after yourself and striving to make healthier choices in your life so that you can feel better, more relaxed and in excellent mental and physical health.

.

Wellness means different things to different people, of course. There are thousands of influencers and self-proclaimed 'health gurus' out there touting the latest wellness trends and pseudoscience, all promising a vast array of too-good-to-believe health benefits. But, at its heart, wellness is about you finding what you enjoy, what fits within your budget and what makes *you* feel great. It's about practising self-care and understanding that loving yourself is just as important as loving others.

> •
> Loving yourself is just as important as loving others.
> •

For some, spending a holiday getting pampered at a luxury spa resort or booking into an intensive Ayurveda program in India is their idea of wellness. Wellness tourism is a fast-growing industry as holidaymakers swap their cocktails for creative therapy and their sightseeing for silent meditation. There are new spa resorts, yoga retreats and detox clinics popping up all over the world that provide plenty of opportunities to not only take a break from the daily grind but also pick up healthy living habits to incorporate at home.

For others, the idea of wellness might be simply finding time to head off for a nature walk or getting out into the ocean for a refreshing swim each morning. The pursuit of health and wellbeing doesn't need to cost a fortune or require you to fly halfway around the world, and you don't have to fundamentally change what you're doing. The important thing to realise is that the basics – fresh air, exercise, healthy eating and reducing stress – are some of the most powerful ways of achieving wellness and self-care. And these are all things you can do at home.

Destination Wellness gives you different ways you can achieve health and wellbeing, from soaking in geothermal waters and indulging in a luxurious massage to enjoying a yoga session and gazing at the stars. Whether it be in the sanctuary of your own home or at one of the many international destinations included here, I hope you find inspiration and ideas to send you off on your own personal wellness journey.

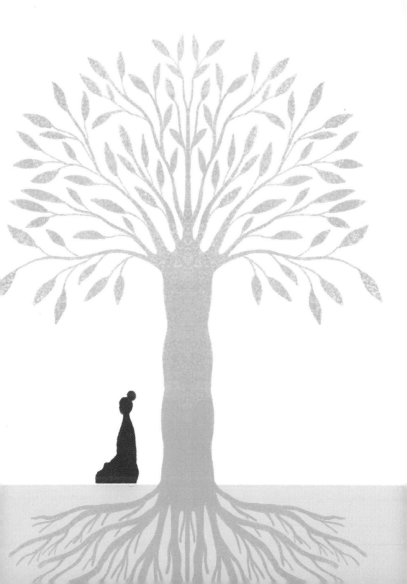

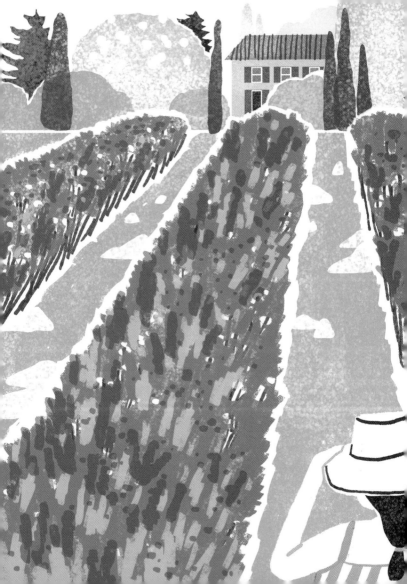

Aromatherapy

How do you feel when you catch the scent of a loved one's perfume or aftershave, smell the fragrance of your favourite flower, get a whiff of the salty ocean air or inhale a waft of your beloved childhood meal cooked by grandma? Smell is an incredibly powerful sense — it can elicit strong emotions and vivid memories — and aromatherapy taps into this olfactory wonder by letting our noses do the healing. Plants and herbs have been used for their potent therapeutic powers for centuries — frankincense and myrrh received notable shout-outs in the Bible — and the practice of aromatherapy harnesses these healing properties to improve an individual's mental and physical wellbeing, working in conjunction with Western medicine.

•

Aromatherapy is essentially the practice of using naturally extracted phytochemicals from medicinal plants and converting them into essential oils for healing and relaxation. Essential oils can be used in a range of ways such as adding drops to scent a bath, mixing into massage oils, using in scented candles or evaporating in oil burners or diffusers. Different oils have their own healing properties and it's important to note that some plants and herbs can be toxic, interfere with medication, be unsafe during pregnancy or have a host of other side-effects, so you need to get expert advice. It's also important to buy quality oils from reputable brands to ensure you're using a pure form that hasn't been loaded with additives and chemicals.

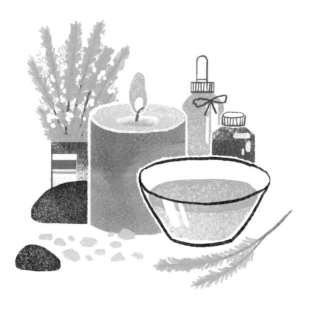

AROMATHERAPY AT HOME

Mix up your own essential oil blends for some at-home aromatherapy sessions. Essential oils are usually blended with what's called a carrier or base oil first as the essential oils are highly concentrated and need to be diluted to avoid any irritation or inflammation. You can use a range of oils for the carrier, including coconut, macadamia, olive or avocado.

There are many books on aromatherapy available but a good one to start with, especially for its recipes, is *Essential Oils and Aromatherapy: An Introductory Guide* published by Sonoma Press.

Massage oil
In a small bottle or container, mix together 20 millilitres of your preferred carrier oil, 4 drops of lavender oil, 4 drops of rosemary oil and 2 drops of ginger oil for an invigorating and muscle-soothing massage.

Bath oil
In a glass dropper bottle, combine 10 drops of lavender, 8 drops of chamomile and 6 drops of sandalwood and shake well. Add 6–8 drops to a warm bath for a relaxing soak.

Pillow spray
To lull yourself into a good night's sleep, add 6–8 drops of essential oils such as lavender, chamomile and rose into 30 millilitres of water in a spray bottle, shake and spray on pillows and sheets before bed.

Grow your own healing herbs

Herbs and plants have been used in healing for centuries to assist with illnesses and ailments — everything from colds and flu to insomnia and muscle pain. Once you know the medicinal properties of different herbs (and which ones can be toxic and should be avoided), you can easily grow them at home in pots or in the garden so you'll have a healing garden at your fingertips for cooking, blending your own herbal tea, making simple herbal remedies or using in aromatherapy. Before using herbs for medicinal purposes, discuss it with your healthcare provider as some herbs can have adverse effects or interfere with certain medications.

·

ALOE VERA

- The clear gel inside the leaves can be used on sunburn, cuts and minor burns.

- It moisturises the skin and may help with acne.

- It's a succulent and prefers the tropics. Grow in full sun outdoors and water occasionally.

GINGER

- The root and ground spice are often used in cooking. Grate the root into a fresh juice or smoothie or make a warming tea with hot water, slices of ginger root and honey.

- Ginger has anti-inflammatory properties, can ease an upset stomach and assists with bloating and nausea.

- It prefers a tropical or subtropical environment. There are many species of ginger so check the specific growing conditions for yours.

CHAMOMILE

- This soothing herb is often served as a tea (which you can make from the dried flowers).

- It's good for digestion and gastrointestinal issues, has a calming, relaxing effect and is great before bed.

- Sow seeds early in spring in a sunny spot.

SAGE

- The fuzzy grey-green leaves are a great aromatic in cooking. Fry the leaves and add to pasta and soups, or use to create marinades and flavoursome sauces.

- Loaded with antioxidants, sage has antibacterial and antifungal properties.

- Infuse sage leaves in hot water and gargle for a sore throat. It helps digestive issues, too.

- Sage is easy to grow and does well in cold and temperate conditions. Plant in full sun.

CINNAMON

- The ground spice, stick and bark are commonly used in cooking; it's delicious sprinkled over porridge or added to smoothies.

- It has antibacterial and antifungal properties, and may reduce blood pressure and inflammation.

- Cinnamon plants eventually mature into trees. It thrives in the tropics and prefers full sun. You can harvest the bark a few years after planting.

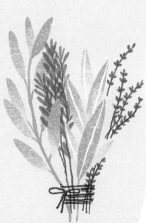

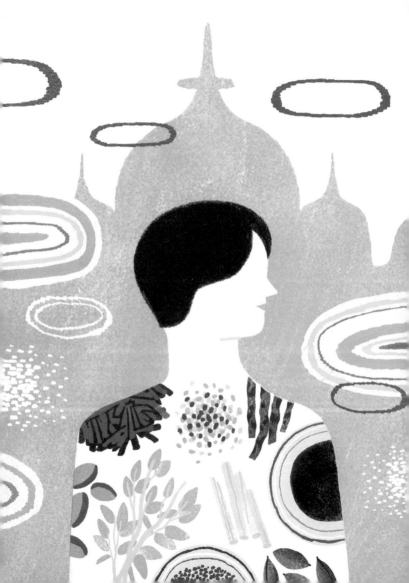

Ayurveda

Ayurveda might sound like a mysterious alternative medicine favoured by hippies and New-Agers, but this ancient healing practice dates back over 5000 years in India. Ayurveda, meaning 'knowledge of life', is the science of Indian herbal medicine and a holistic approach to health and wellbeing. It focuses on restoring balance in the body and centres on the mind–body connection — what's good for the mind is good for the body and vice versa. It's still widely practised in India today and is becoming increasingly popular around the world as people strive to get back in tune with the body and mind to heal from the stresses of modern life.

.

According to Ayurvedic principles, the key to overall health and wellbeing is to have a well-functioning digestive system and maintain balance in the body. It's not a one-size-fits-all science though; everyone is different and no single treatment, program or remedy will work for everyone. Ayurveda specifies three mind–body types, or 'doshas', that are present in everyone.

The three doshas are vata, pitta and kapha. Vata relates to the movement of the body (gastrointestinal, circulation, breathing), pitta relates to the metabolic system (digestion, temperature, metabolism) and kapha relates to the body's structure (fat regulation, muscle strength, bone density). People have all three doshas but one is usually dominant; an Ayurveda practitioner will work with you to find out which dosha is your dominant one and then outline a treatment plan to remedy any energy imbalances through diet, herbal remedies and massage.

WHAT'S SO GOOD ABOUT IT?

Since Ayurveda is a holistic practice, it offers benefits not just for your body but also for your mind and your spiritual self. It aims to restore balance and also teaches you to slow down and listen to your body, to become more in tune with what's going on and how you're feeling. Ayurvedic treatments are used to help with a range of ailments including digestive problems, anxiety, stress, inflammation and asthma. If you'd like to find out more, pick up one of the many fascinating books on the subject, such as Sahara Rose Ketabi's *Ayurveda*.

WHERE IN THE WORLD CAN I TRY IT?

India

The birthplace of Ayurveda, India is home to countless Ayurveda centres, resorts and practitioners ranging from reputable to questionable and from budget to ludicrous. Somatheeram, located by the sea, is one of the best Ayurveda resorts in the Kerala region. The luxurious Ananda Spa, located in the Himalayas, offers the Ayurveda Rejuvenation Programme, which is tailored to your needs, while Ayuskama Ayurvedic Clinic is another well-respected centre in Bhagsu near Rishikesh.

Austria

Located in the ridiculously scenic Tyrolean Alps in Austria is one of Europe's finest Ayurveda resorts, the Sonnhof. Expert practitioners determine your dosha before guiding you through a host of treatments and therapies from acupuncture, chakra-cleansing and meditation to yoga, deep-tissue massage and soothing shirodhara, where warm oil is poured in a continuous flow across your forehead.

Germany

Founded in the early 1990s by the late Wolfgang Preuss, Ayurveda Parkschlösschen is a five-star Ayurveda resort located in peaceful woodland. A team of highly qualified staff customise treatments to suit your needs. The retreat specialises in Panchakarma cures, an intensive detox program over 9, 13, 20 or 34 nights. Wake up with tongue scraping and oil pulling followed by yoga, massage, meditation and exceptionally tasty Ayurvedic cuisine.

Ayurveda aims to restore balance and teaches you to become more in tune with how you're feeling.

START YOUR DAY RIGHT

According to Ayurveda, if you start your morning right, the rest of the day will follow suit. So, instead of snoozing late, buzzing off a couple of coffees and scoffing down some toast, why not take an Ayurvedic approach with a few morning rituals?

Tongue scraping

Our teeth are surely the envy of our tongue, getting all the brushing attention and care every morning while the tongue is neglected. In Ayurveda, a gentle tongue scraping when you wake up is considered an essential task to remove toxic build-up from the mouth and to help eliminate bad breath. A U-shaped copper scraper is the tool of choice as using your toothbrush won't remove bacteria and toxins completely.

Oil pulling

What is the first thing you feel like doing as soon as you wake up? Rinsing out your mouth with a good dose of oil? Yep, that's what I thought – a resounding no. As distasteful as it sounds, though, Ayurveda suggests that oil pulling (basically using a natural oil such as coconut, sesame or olive as a mouthwash for about 20 minutes) can help to remove toxins and promote better oral health. Ensure you avoid swallowing any oil and don't forget to spit it all out.

Dry brushing

After you've taken care of your oral hygiene, rid your body of its toxins, boost circulation and remove dead skin cells with a short bout of dry brushing. This is best done before you shower. With a natural-bristled brush (you can easily find these online or at beauty stores and pharmacies) and starting at your feet, make long, gentle yet firm brush strokes towards your heart and work your way up your body. Hop in the shower to rinse off afterwards and then apply moisturiser. Do this a couple of times a week.

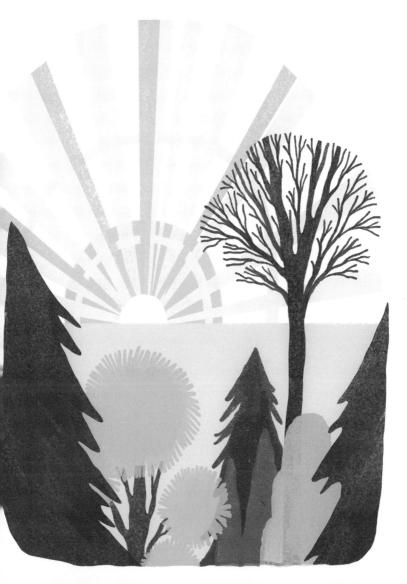

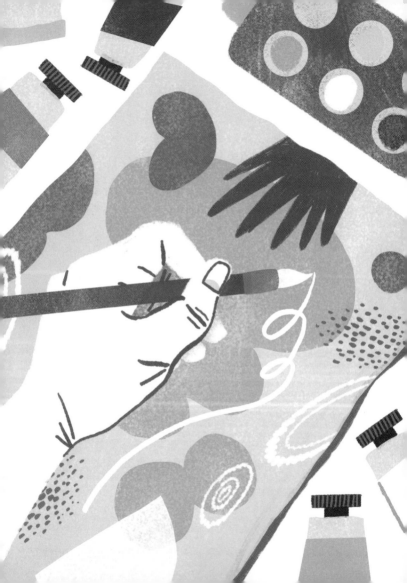

Creative therapy

When it comes to creativity, some people are fortunate enough to have it running through their veins. They simply pick up a paintbrush, a camera or a guitar and are able to produce a masterpiece. While we can't all be Picasso, Man Ray or Jimi Hendrix, we all have the ability to express ourselves through art and creative pursuits, and the end result is not what matters.

Many of us take to creativity simply for pleasure and enjoyment, but these activities can also be extremely beneficial for our mental wellbeing. Whether you're into painting, drawing, writing, photography or playing the banjo, dedicating time to these activities on a daily basis can help you relax and reduce stress. For those suffering from more severe mental health issues, creative therapy or art therapy can be practised in guided sessions with licensed practitioners.

FIND YOUR INNER CREATIVITY

If you don't consider yourself a creative person and the idea of trying to paint a landscape, learn the piano or write a poem is overwhelming, remember creativity comes in many forms. You might prefer knitting, gardening, cooking a dish you've never tried before or trying your hand at pottery – all are creative undertakings. Even the simple act of colouring in can be therapeutic and it's no longer just for kids; many adult colouring books are available for meditation and relaxation purposes.

WHAT'S SO GOOD ABOUT IT?

When we engage in a creative activity we enjoy, the brain releases dopamine, a chemical that helps us feel good. It can have a significant therapeutic effect on the mind and body, akin to being in a meditative state, as it helps focus our attention on one activity. You can't drift off into worrying about the future or ruminating on the past when you are totally in the moment with an enthralling creative project. It keeps your mind calm and focused.

This experience of focus is often referred to as 'flow', a state where your concentration takes over and you're completely absorbed without any effort. Therefore, creative activities can be incredibly beneficial for those suffering from anxiety, depression and other mental health issues. Immersing yourself in a creative activity is a great way of disconnecting your mind from stress; it allows you to have a break and escape from your worries for a time.

Creative therapy can help with a range of issues including depression and post-traumatic stress disorder (PTSD). When we are preoccupied with negative thoughts and emotions, channelling those into something positive through creativity can be cathartic and healing. If you feel uncomfortable or unable to talk about stressful situations or memories, creative therapy is a way of overcoming this barrier to healing. Journalling, painting and drawing are often easier ways to truly express emotion and trauma. Creative activities also require us to slow down, reflect on how we're feeling and perhaps see our world in a new light.

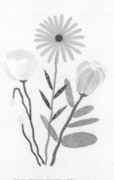

Paris Writers' Retreat, France

Paris's cobblestoned streets and cafe terraces are packed with hopeful writers scribbling notes in their Moleskins, lured in by the rich history and romance of the City of Lights. It's no surprise then that there are countless writing courses and workshops available in the city, but the Paris Writers' Retreat, held in a gorgeous loft space, is the standout bestseller among them. Run by *New York Times* bestselling author and literary agent Wendy Goldman Rohm, this retreat attracts serious writers for its five-day intensive course where you learn about the nuances of the writing craft from some of the most talented literary names in the business. Hopefully by the end you'll be armed with enough guidance and inspiration to finally finish that novel. Bonne chance!

National Geographic photography workshops, global

If you're serious about improving your photography skills and want to team it with a holiday, *National Geographic* hosts a range of photography workshops in remote locations around the world, from the wilds of Alaska to the magnificent Galápagos Islands. You'll get hands-on instruction from a *National Geographic* photographer and plenty of chances to take some incredible shots.

Omega Institute, United States

Set in the heart of New York's Hudson Valley hills, the Omega Institute has been guiding people on creative journeys since 1977. This holistic haven runs retreats featuring an abundance of creative workshops, in addition to its social workshops and wellness treatments. It also offers workshops online. Find out how to unleash your creativity, learn the art of watercolour painting or craft a piece of writing, to name just a few of the Institute's fabulous creative opportunities.

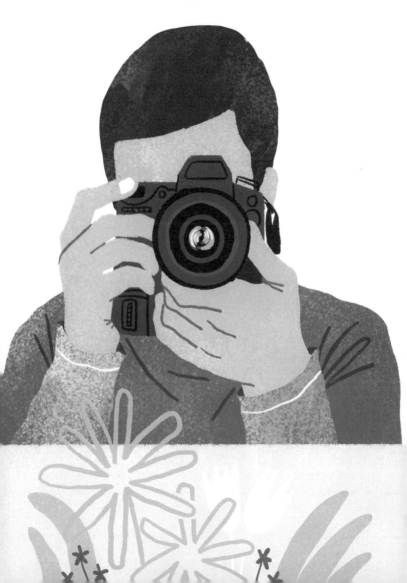

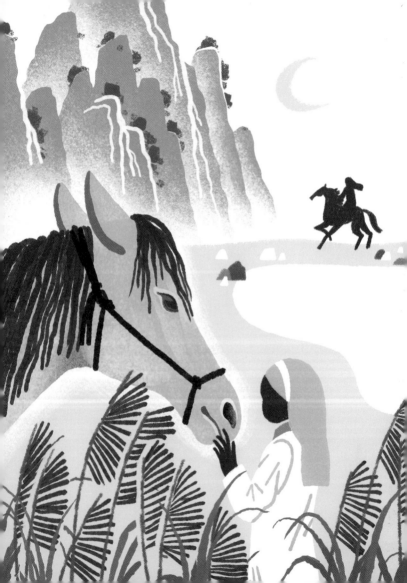

Equine therapy

Animals help humans in countless ways and we rely on our four-legged, two-legged, no-legged, furry, scaly, aquatic friends for a variety of reasons. Beloved pets provide companionship, specially trained service dogs provide an important support for vision-impaired individuals and those who require mobility assistance, and you can even have a goat sidekick at your yoga sessions these days. And if you're in need of emotional support, comfort and affection, therapy animals have got your back.

•

Therapy animals are specifically trained to provide support for people suffering from a range of health issues including stress, anxiety, PTSD, low self-esteem and trauma. Dogs are the most common therapy animal and these fluffy visitors put a smile on the faces of people in hospitals, aged-care facilities and schools. While dogs might be the most popular choice of therapy animal, horses are becoming more widely used in this area of wellness and mental health in what is known as equine therapy or equine-assisted therapy. Sure, Mr Ed won't be hopping onto any laps for a pat and a chat any time soon, but these intuitive animals are providing their services at dedicated equine therapy centres, working alongside qualified mental health practitioners in guided sessions to help lead people on a journey of self-discovery and healing.

Horses are large and imposing, weigh a truckload and can be very intimidating, but in the right environment with trained professionals safely guiding the process, we can work together with horses to develop a bond, build deep trust and feel safe in each other's presence. As horses are known to be highly perceptive, they can mirror what might be going on in our lives; this can help bring our issues and emotions to the surface so we can work on them.

WHAT'S SO GOOD ABOUT IT?

You can lead a horse to water but you can't make it cure your crippling anxiety, low self-esteem or past trauma. Or can you? It's thought that horses have a natural ability to create a calming and nurturing environment; they are perceptive to emotions, sensitive to movement and able to pick up on body language cues, which makes them effective in therapy.

Each equine therapy session is created to meet an individual's specific needs and might include grooming, petting and feeding a horse, companion-walking side-by-side or simply spending time bonding. It rarely involves any actual horse-riding.

Both adults and children can take part in equine therapy and it has been used to help teens with bullying, low self-esteem and low confidence. As Sandra Jelly from Pink Spirit retreats says, 'Horses "see" you for all that you are, they bring you back into the present moment of pure love and divine potential. The true place from where you can heal, transform reality and manifest your dreams.'

> Horses 'see' you for all that you are, they bring you back into the present moment of pure love and divine potential.

Jordan

Picture yourself in Jordan's Wadi Rum region, warm breeze floating over you, horse nuzzling into your side as the dusky pink sun melts into the desert sands. That's exactly the kind of magical experience that awaits at Pink Spirit, where Netherlands-born Sandra Jelly runs guided 'horse soul sessions' in the desert, as part of a retreat including meditation, sacred dance and yoga.

United States

Koelle Simpson is one of the most highly regarded 'horse whisperers' in the world and is the founder of the Koelle Institute for Equus Coaching, set on a sprawling ranch in Central California. Her equine coaching sessions are a journey of personal transformation where the horse is considered the teacher. You can book private or group sessions or, to simply observe the process, there are live sessions held regularly where you have the opportunity to watch a trained coach demonstrate how the horse's behaviour assists the participants' self-discovery.

New Zealand

The native bush and serene countryside of New Zealand set the scene for healing at Vanora. This company is certified by the Equine Assisted Growing and Learning Association and is located half an hour north of Dunedin. Vanora's mental health professionals safely guide clients in equine-assisted therapy to help with everything from abuse, depression and addiction to eating disorders and PTSD.

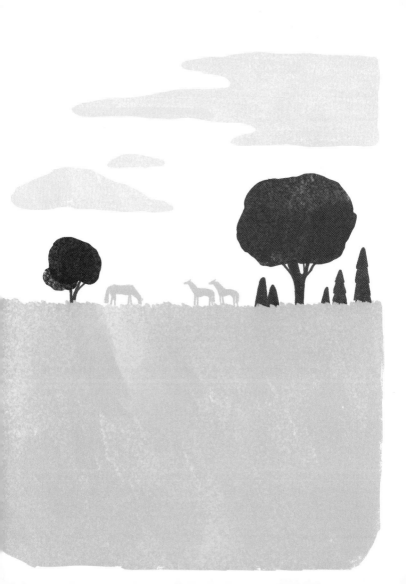

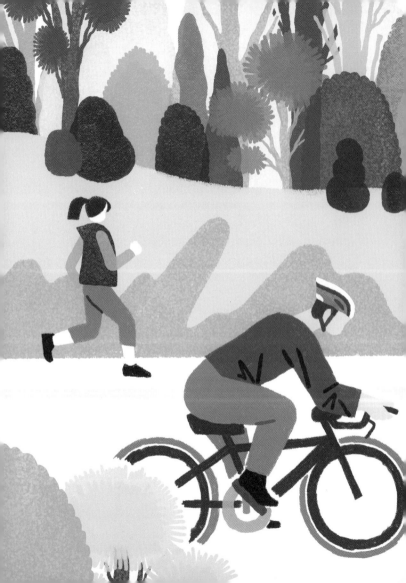

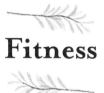

Fitness

It's no secret that being active and keeping fit leads to a healthier and happier life, and you don't have to pump iron like The Rock to get there. If you're not much of a gym bunny, head outdoors where there are myriad ways to stay fit, from hiking, skiing and surfing to stand-up paddleboarding, swimming and cycling. Take the time to find a fitness activity you actually enjoy as you'll have more success in sticking with it and achieving your goals.

.

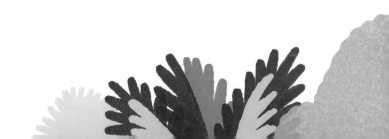

The first step is assessing your fitness level so you know where to start. If you haven't been on a regular fitness program or are new to exercising or a particular activity, it's important to ease into it; motivation and enthusiasm peak at the start of a fitness kick but if you go out all muscles blazing it's a good way to get injured, burn out that enthusiasm and be right back on the couch before you know it. Most government dietary guidelines recommend that adults do at least two to five hours of moderate-intensity physical activity each week to maintain a healthy weight, so that's a good goal to start with if you're new to exercise.

Approaching your fitness program with a healthy attitude is also crucial – don't set yourself unrealistic goals of extreme weight loss or spending hours and hours each day exercising. Balance is the key and you need to factor in recovery so your body has time to rest between exercise sessions. And listen to your body. The popular 1980s slogan 'No pain, no gain' is about as on point today as Walkmans and shoulder pads. If you feel pain, take a break.

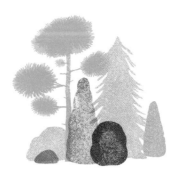

One of the best things about physical activity is it releases endorphins and gives you an overall improved feeling of wellbeing, even if at first you feel sweaty, exhausted and ready to give up. It can relieve symptoms of anxiety, stress and depression, too. Research shows that engaging in regular physical activity boosts your stamina, strength, flexibility and energy and can help you lose weight, get a better night's sleep and keep the doctor away by improving cardiovascular health, boosting blood flow and lowering blood pressure.

KEEP FIT AT HOME

If heading outdoors or to the gym is not an option for you, take your workout online where you can find thousands of fitness 'gurus' guiding classes in everything from yoga (*see* p. 96 for some easy at-home yoga poses) and high-intensity interval training (HIIT) to Pilates, boxing and dance workouts favoured by A-list celebs. A number of gyms also offer online access to at-home workouts with personal trainers. Otherwise, order yourself some budget workout equipment such as dumbbells, a fit ball, resistance bands and a skipping rope and get to work.

Aro Ha, New Zealand

Overlooking Lake Wakatipu, Aro Ha is a luxury health and fitness resort in an alpine wilderness just under an hour from Queenstown. The strict no alcohol, meat, sugar, gluten and dairy restrictions might have you uninspired and overwhelmed at first but the spectacular mountain views will definitely perk you up ready to begin your journey on the path to a fitter, healthier you. That journey starts with a yoga session and a sub-alpine 10–15-kilometre (6–9-mile) hike – all before lunch – followed by strength training, perhaps some Pilates and more yoga to end the day. Don't worry, there is downtime in between for relaxing massages, rejuvenating spa treatments and nutritional cooking demos.

Canyon Ranch, United States

An icon of the wellness industry in the United States, Canyon Ranch has been inspiring people to lead fitter, healthier and more spiritual lives since it opened its first retreat in 1979 in the Santa Catalina Mountains in Tucson, Arizona. Daily activities are packed in and range from group hikes and back-country cycling to rock climbing, yoga and ziplining. There are four pools to choose from and an extensive menu of indulgent spa treatments to enjoy once the hard work is done.

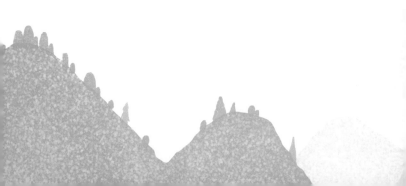

Wildfitness, global

Founded in 2001 by Kenyan-born Tara Wood, Wildfitness holds retreats in a variety of destinations around the world, from Costa Rica and Crete to Iceland and Menorca, and is based on the vision, 'To help anyone rediscover the joy and transformative power of their own natural potential'. Groups are kept intimate at 8 to 12 people and, while physical activities are challenging and gruelling, they are kept fun and varied and cater to all fitness levels. You might find yourself hiking up a mountain one minute, then catching some waves on a surfboard the next, before taking in a few rounds of boxing in the beautiful outdoors. The retreats aim to provide you with tools to incorporate what you learn into your life back home.

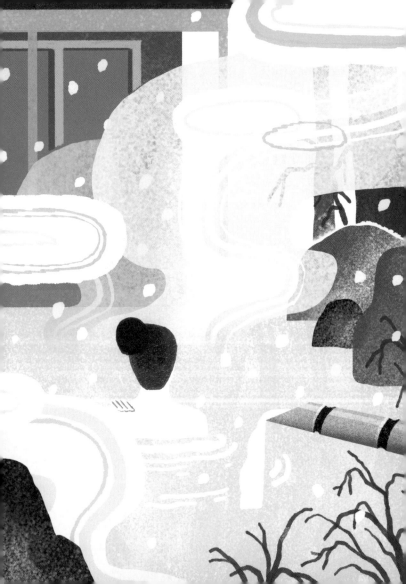

Geothermal bathing

For many of us, the idea of taking a long soak in
a hot bath is the stuff of pure relaxation dreams
where we can soothe aching muscles, release body
tension and drift off to our happy place. For others,
however, a bath is the stuff of nightmares — akin to
marinating in a cesspool of your own bacteria. If you
don't happen to be a fan of submerging yourself in
tap water at home, geothermal bathing in hot springs
might be more up your alley, with all its mineral
goodness and bacteria-killing scorching temperatures
(as long as you don't have a strong aversion to the
smell of rotten eggs, that is).

•

Hot springs, or thermal pools, usually form when water deep below the Earth's surface is heated by magma. This creates steam and hot water, which rises to the surface through cracks and fissures in the ground, forming pools. That's why hot springs are generally found in areas of either active volcanos, where the water is way too hot for humans, or in inactive volcanic regions, where the water temperature is between 37°C (98.6°F) and 42°C (107.6°F) – perfect for a nice hot soak.

WHAT'S SO GOOD ABOUT IT?

Bathing in geothermal waters is an age-old tradition and these waters are believed to have curative properties thanks to their high mineral content. Minerals commonly found in hot springs include magnesium, zinc, potassium and sulphate, along with the olfactory delight that is hydrogen sulphide (that rotten-egg smell). The reported therapeutic benefits of geothermal bathing range from improving sleep and aiding relaxation to boosting blood circulation and helping skin conditions such as eczema.

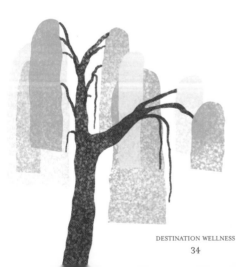

Japan

Hot springs, ubiquitous in Japan, are known as onsen and are an integral part of Japanese culture. Situated in the Pacific Ring of Fire, Japan is literally bubbling with volcanic activity and many parts of the country are misted over with rising steam from the many hot springs. Often, ryokan (traditional lodgings) have their own on-site onsen – you can enjoy a heavenly pre-bedtime soak. Rotenburo (open-air onsen), many with scenic mountain or ocean views, offer a serene experience or simply an opportunity for stargazing in the evening. Naked communal bathing is what onsen are all about (usually gender-segregated), so leaving your inhibitions at home is the first step.

It's tough to pick the best onsen in Japan with so many to choose from, but a great place to start is Kinosaki, a charming town that seems to be lifted straight from a Japanese woodblock print, with weeping willows dangling over pretty canals and the choice of seven onsen to experience. Another standout, Dōgo Onsen, in Matsuyama, is one of the oldest and best known onsen in the country; the main building here dates back to 1894. It's undergoing a major renovation, expected to be completed in 2026, but sections are still open to the public. And the setting at Takaragawa Onsen couldn't be more serene; the large outdoor onsen sits alongside Takaragawa River, shaded by forest and surrounded by mountains in the Gunma prefecture.

Iceland

While its name might suggest otherwise, Iceland is another hotbed (sorry, but pun intended) of volcanic activity and the cool temperature outside makes splashing around in geothermal pools, or 'hot pots' as they're known locally, extremely enticing and a hugely popular pastime for locals. The Blue Lagoon, in Iceland's south-west, is the star of the show, but there are plenty more steamy spots, including Mývatn Nature Baths located in the north, where steam rises from the mineral-loaded waters amid a sci-fi volcanic landscape, and Krossneslaug, a 'hot pot' infinity pool set on a black-pebbled beachfront where you can take in the views of the lapping Arctic waters.

Turkey

It would be remiss not to mention Turkey's famed Pamukkale as one of the best places in the world for geothermal bathing. Listed as a World Heritage site and located by the ruins of the ancient Roman city of Hierapolis, these stunning white, chalky calcite formations of natural terraced pools have been easing physical ailments for millennia. Let the warm mineral-rich waters soothe your muscles while you take in the incredible mountain views.

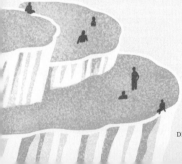

ONSEN ETIQUETTE

Bathing in an onsen for the first time can be daunting for a tourist in Japan but it's nothing to get your knickers in a knot about (you'll need to take them off anyway). Your best bet is to follow the locals' lead and do what they do, but these pointers will help.

Head into the change room and get your gear off, all of it, and pop your belongings in a locker. If you'd like a little bit of privacy, you can usually hire hand towels for a small fee.

Wash before you bathe. It might sound a little backward but it actually makes complete sense. At most onsen you'll find a row of shower taps and stools. Sit down, lather up and wash yourself diligently before rinsing off thoroughly.

Slide into the onsen and relax. The water can get very hot so be sure to take a break if you feel light-headed. To cool off a little, you can rinse your towel in cold water and pop it on your head as the locals often do.

Some onsen refuse entry to tattooed folk (tattoos being associated with the yakuza, the Japanese mafia) so, if you're inked, it's best to check beforehand.

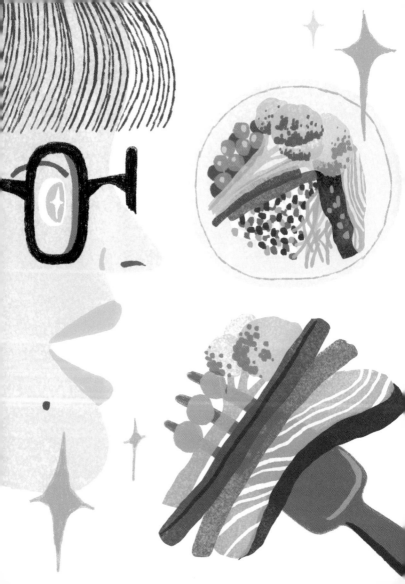

Healthy eating

Should I swap my morning coffee for a green
smoothie or matcha tea? Or should I stick to an all-
ancient-grain diet? Carbs are evil, dairy is the devil's
work and even cooking your food is so 2010 now that
raw is all the rage. With so much information and
misinformation about what we should and shouldn't
be eating these days, it's challenging to know how to
make sense of it all. Where do you begin?

•

One minute you're stocking your fridge full of kale, the next you're working out what end of a kohlrabi you should be eating and trying to grow your own alien-like scoby for homemade kombucha. And then there's the minefield of fad diets out there spruiked by celebrities – everything from keto and paleo to juice cleansing and only eating foods that suit your blood type. In reality, many of these diets can be downright dangerous or, at the very least, not sustainable.

Essentially, the key to healthy eating is keeping your diet balanced: nourish yourself with lots of fruit and veg, wholegrains, healthy fats, nuts and lean protein (favouring fish and poultry over red meat) and cut back on too much sugar. But it's also important to enjoy a little treat every now and then. Qualified nutritionists and dieticians can help you make sense of it all and cut through the noise with dedicated expert advice. They can educate you on how to eat healthily and will also devise an individualised program for you to follow.

WHAT'S SO GOOD ABOUT IT?

It makes sense that what you choose to eat will directly affect how you feel, from your energy levels and your mood to your weight. If you make healthy food choices, you can reduce your risk of ailments such as heart disease, inflammation, cancer and digestive issues, and significantly improve the quality of your physical, mental and emotional wellbeing. Try the following steps on your journey to eating well and feeling well.

Manage portion size

We've all done it: you cook a big load of pasta or curry and think you'll keep the leftovers for lunch tomorrow, but as soon as you've wolfed down your meal you're back loading up seconds and tomorrow's lunch is tomorrow's problem. Limiting portion sizes is crucial in healthy eating; a great tip is to stop eating when you feel about 80 per cent full, rather than eating until you feel completely full.

Try to eat in-season produce

Eating produce when it's in season means you're eating fresh food, and research shows that it's usually more nutrient dense when compared with out-of-season produce. In-season, fresh produce also tends to taste a whole lot better, and if you're buying locally grown fruit and veg you're also helping the environment by cutting down on food miles. Win-win.

Go organic if possible

I'm sure many of us would love to switch to an all-organic diet but sometimes it's simply not in our budget. Growing evidence suggests an organic diet is a healthier choice as you're consuming fewer harmful pesticides, synthetic hormones, antibiotics and heavy metals. So, if you do have the means to go organic, it's a wise decision. If your budget doesn't stretch to an all-organic diet, try swapping the main offenders – some studies show that strawberries, potatoes and spinach are among the fruit and veg that contain high levels of pesticides.

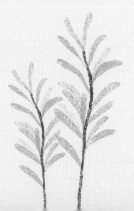

The Mediterranean

Known to be one of the world's healthiest diets, the Mediterranean approach to eating generally involves an abundance of fresh seasonal produce, wholefoods, extra virgin olive oil, seafood and plenty of nuts. Red meat, dairy, salt and sugar are consumed in limited amounts. Numerous studies over the years have found that the Mediterranean diet is good for the heart and can help reduce the risk of heart disease, dementia, type 2 diabetes and high cholesterol. And, best of all, by following the Mediterranean diet you don't have to feel guilty about a glass or two of red wine. Cheers to that.

Japan

Sushi is becoming an increasingly popular go-to healthy lunch or dinner option not only for its convenience but also for its health benefits. The Japanese diet has long been considered a healthy one, rich in fermented foods, grains and fresh seafood with minimal dairy, sugar and refined foods. Japan has one of the highest life-expectancy rates in the world and some of the lowest obesity rates. In fact, the Okinawa islands, in Japan's south, have some of the highest numbers of centenarians in the world, which has been partly attributed to their diet. The traditional Okinawan diet features modest amounts of fish rich in omega-3 fatty acids, plenty of fresh vegetables such as sweet potato and leafy greens, soy products and wholefoods. So you might want to start choosing Japanese for lunch more often.

Nordic countries

Traditionally, the Scandinavian countries of Denmark, Sweden, Finland, Norway and Iceland have a diet rich in oily fish, root vegetables and wholegrain bread, making it a high-fibre, high-protein, low-sugar diet that rivals the Mediterranean as one of the reported healthiest diets around. The protein mainly comes from seafood, and meat and dairy are eaten in minimal quantities. The Nordic diet is based on fresh, seasonal and sustainably sourced ingredients, limits the amount of processed foods consumed and incorporates fermented foods into meals – great for gut health.

RETREATS FOR HEALTHY EATING

If you're looking to make some healthy changes to your diet but don't know where to start, there are plenty of great health and nutrition retreats around the world where you can learn about everything from gut health and fermenting your own food at home to recipes for healthy snacks and how to grown your own veggies.

Gwinganna Lifestyle Retreat, Australia

This luxurious award-winning eco-retreat is located among the forested mountains of Australia's Gold Coast hinterland and invites you to leave your distractions (including coffee, alcohol and cigarettes) at the door and step into an exclusive world of wellness. Nutritional, seasonal, organic wholefoods make up the cuisine with most ingredients sourced from the on-site garden, and there's no gluten or dairy in sight. Retreat packages offer food-focused options where you can learn how to grow your own organic veggies or discover the secrets of superfoods with a clinical nutritionist.

The Farm at San Benito, the Philippines

A much-needed respite from Manila's frenetic pace, the Farm at San Benito is hidden away in lush jungle a two-hour drive from the capital and is a firm favourite of celebs in need of some time out. The Farm's award-winning vegan restaurant, Alive!, will have you feeling just that after you've tucked into its tasty dishes made using organic produce from the retreat's garden. Methods such as dehydration and fermentation are employed to ensure maximum nutritional value in the cooking. If you prefer a little something from the sea to pep up your plate, the retreat's Pesce restaurant serves only wild-caught seafood.

SHA Wellness Clinic, Spain

The SHA Wellness Clinic, located on the edge of the Mediterranean Sea, offers an extensive list of treatments and tailored programs with a focus on nutrition. As you would expect, the cuisine at SHA is all organic, seasonal and healthy, and there are three delicious menus to choose from depending on how strict you're wanting to go. The Chef's Studio is where you'll learn some of the retreat's recipe secrets and ways to clean up your diet once home.

Stock up on superfoods

Not a day goes by without yet another article or
social media post raving about the latest superfood.
One moment chia seeds and goji berries are all on
trend, the next people are adding açaí powder to
every meal, activating their almonds and overdosing
on kefir. Marketing claims have superfoods curing
everything from cancer to high cholesterol, but
in reality there's no silver bullet and it's best to
avoid trends. Instead, for long-term wellness and
abundant health, strive to eat more of the foods
that are high in essential vitamins and nutrients.
Here are some of the best.

.

DARK LEAFY GREENS

Think kale, spinach and silverbeet. They're packed with fibre, minerals and vitamins A, C and K. Eat them raw in salad, sauté and add to pasta or soup, or include in a tasty omelette.

BERRIES

Another antioxidant-rich food source, berries are also high in fibre and low in calories. Try adding blueberries to your morning muesli or enjoy raspberries or strawberries with some yoghurt when you need a healthy and delicious pick-me-up.

GREEN TEA

Next time you go to make a cup of black tea or coffee try switching for a cup of green tea. There are plenty of varieties of green tea, and Japanese matcha (powdered green tea) is an excellent choice. While it's still high in caffeine, it doesn't usually produce caffeine's typical jittery side-effects thanks to the amino acid L-theanine, which slows the release of caffeine. It's also high in antioxidants.

DARK CHOCOLATE

You can still satisfy your sweet tooth when following a healthy balanced diet. Dark chocolate is a great choice as it contains flavonoids (powerful antioxidants) and has less sugar than milk chocolate. Opt for at least 70 per cent cacao for the most health benefits.

OILY FISH

Oily fish such as salmon, sardines and mackerel are rich in omega-3 fatty acids, which have the potential to reduce the risk of heart disease and certain cancers.

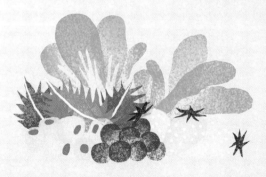

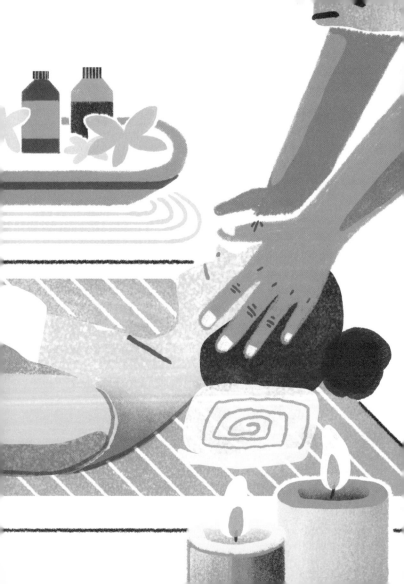

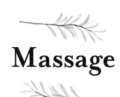

Massage

Massage therapy is thought to be one of the oldest healing traditions in the world and has been used as a therapeutic practice for thousands of years. While there are some standard classic massage styles – Swedish, shiatsu, Thai – the practice is ever-evolving. These days you can opt for a physio-style sports massage at a health clinic, go first class with sandalwood-scented oil at a luxury day spa or even get a quick lunchtime rub-down by an on-site masseuse in your office.

•

Whether you like your kidneys pummelled, your pressure points poked at, the feel of hot smooth stones weighing on your back or strong hands gently kneading your muscle tension away, there is a massage style for you. Often your preference will depend on the reason for getting one in the first place: are you after an hour of total body relaxation or do you need your deep tissue seen to after an injury?

Basically, massage is the manual manipulation (rubbing, kneading and, yes, sometimes what feels like torturing) of a person's muscles and soft tissue in order to improve health and wellbeing and assist in the prevention or treatment of certain ailments.

WHAT'S SO GOOD ABOUT IT?

You know that dreamy, floating feeling after a massage? It's thanks to the fact that massage therapy releases endorphins, those feel-good brain chemicals that help us feel calm and relaxed. As well as inducing relaxation and reducing stress levels, massage offers a host of other benefits ranging from reduced pain and muscle tension to a stronger immune system, depending on the style of the therapy and amount of pressure applied. Studies suggest that regular massage can help with pain management as it loosens stiff muscles and increases blood circulation. This can also help increase flexibility and work as a preventative measure against injuries. By alleviating stress in the body, massage can boost the immune system to help fight off infections and illnesses.

YOUR MASSAGE MENU

Like many wellness modalities, massage trends come and
go. There are many styles available, some common with
well-studied benefits – Swedish, deep tissue, relaxation –
and some more 'out there' (with less evidence of efficacy).
It's worth doing your research and speaking with your
doctor, especially before choosing one of the lesser known
styles. Here are some of the many massage styles you
will see available:

- bodywork
- Burmese
- craniosacral
- cupping
- deep tissue
- hot stone
- lomilomi
- lymphatic drainage
- myofascial release

- pregnancy
- reflexology
- relaxation
- rolfing
- shiatsu
- sports
- Swedish
- Thai
- trigger point.

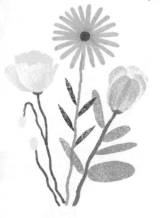

Sweden

When we think of a classic massage, Swedish massage is the type most people think of in the West. If you're new to massage, the Swedish style is a great place to start as it's relaxing and uses long, gliding strokes with some kneading of muscles and friction to stimulate circulation and relieve tight muscles. If you're going to try just one spa in Sweden, make it the historic and opulent Sturebadet in Stockholm. It's long been a favourite haunt of the famous, including Greta Garbo, and offers classic Swedish massages.

Hawaii

If you prefer a more restorative and nurturing style of massage, the traditional Hawaiian massage lomilomi (meaning 'loving hands') is the one for you. This Hawaiian form of healing involves long, sweeping strokes using the hands and forearms, some chanting and the techniques of deep-tissue massage. One of the best places to experience a truly authentic lomilomi massage is at Angeline's Lomi in Anahola on Kauai.

Thailand

If you've only ever had a classic relaxing style of massage and are thinking, 'You know what, I might try a nice Thai one next time', be sure to do your research first! Thai massage has been practised for thousands of years but it's not for the faint of heart – be prepared for your limbs to be pulled, yanked and stretched as you flail around like an inflatable prop at a car sales yard. And your masseuse will treat your pressure points like ancient typewriter keys, pushing in hard all in the name of promoting your internal health. You'll likely leave a little tender, but wonderfully energised.

Health Land in Bangkok is a good-value option for Thai massages by highly trained staff. If you prefer to get semi-tortured in plusher surrounds, the spa at Bangkok's premier hotel, the Mandarin Oriental, is the pinnacle of indulgence.

Japan

One of the most popular massage styles today is shiatsu, an ancient Japanese technique that aims to relieve blockages in the body's energy flow. Based on acupuncture, shiatsu uses finger pressure applied to pressure points along the meridian lines and, while it can feel tender, the aim is for you to feel relaxed while also invigorated.

Set in a beautiful traditional house in Kyoto with private tatami-mat treatment rooms, Hiyoshido is a stellar choice for a top-notch shiatsu massage to work out the knots and relieve muscle fatigue from a busy day of sightseeing. For massage with a touch of high-end sophistication, head to the Four Seasons Tokyo at Marunouchi where you can order room-service shiatsu.

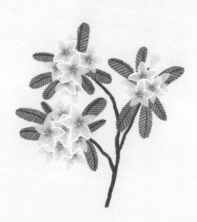

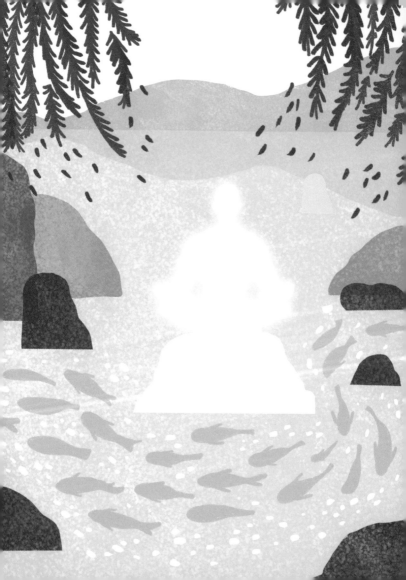

Meditation

The stresses of the modern world can take a real toll on your physical, emotional and mental wellbeing. It's easy to get caught up in daily tasks, work, bumper-to-bumper traffic, delayed trains home, caregiving and domestic duties. On top of this, time seems to vanish as we plunge ourselves into digital rabbit hole after rabbit hole on social media and get lost in a vortex of unrelenting news channels. It's essential to find an escape from the hamster wheel of this life at times. That's where meditation comes in.

.

This mindfulness practice is, of course, nothing new – some archaeologists date its origin to over 2600 years ago in India – and it is deeply rooted in religion, particularly Hinduism and Buddhism. More and more people around the world are now starting to realise that a daily meditation practice can significantly improve mental and physical health and wellbeing. There are loads of different styles of meditation, from vipassana (a self-awareness and insight meditation), chanting mantras and breath awareness to zazen (seated Buddhist zen meditation) and mandala colouring, so you just need to see what works best for you and try to incorporate a daily session into your routine.

WHAT'S SO GOOD ABOUT IT?

Meditation can be a valuable tool in finding a much-needed break from the non-stop inner chatter, clearing the mental clutter and bringing the mind back to the self. When practised regularly, it trains the brain and the nervous system to be present in the moment. When you're present in the moment, you stop worrying about things in the past or uncontrollable events in the future. Meditation provides you with useful tools to manage difficult situations, alleviates stress and anxiety, improves sleep, boosts the immune system and improves concentration.

SAVOUR THE SILENCE

When the everyday noise of beeping smartphones, children's tantrums, roaring traffic and blaring TVs all gets a little too much, seek out silence and solitude at a dedicated silent meditation retreat. These retreats give you the chance to reconnect with your thoughts and feelings for a few days to a few weeks, depending on how noisy your world has become. You take a vow of silence for the dedicated time; the only talking allowed is usually in brief catch-up meetings with retreat guides. Vices such as alcohol, smoking and phones are restricted; by removing all distractions you have only your thoughts, struggles, bodily sensations and emotions to keep you occupied, and this inward focus promotes deep contemplation and personal reflection. Silent meditation is thought to build resilience, help the brain function more effectively and boost overall mental and physical wellbeing.

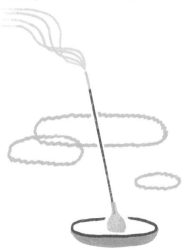

Japan

Buddhism was introduced to Japan in the 6th century and over time several sects were formed, zen being the most well known around the world. Zen meditation is notable for its seated practice (zazen), which involves sitting on a cushion on the floor, paying close attention to the breath and clearing the mind by letting go of any thoughts that arise. It aims to calm the mind and also ultimately offer a path to a deeper spiritual awakening. If you're keen to discover more about zen meditation, read Shunmyō Masuno's *Zen: The Art of Simple Living*.

Japan's iconic zen gardens, known as kare-sansui (dry landscape gardens), are a prominent feature of zen meditation and provide contemplative spots to practise. The best place to see these gardens with their carefully raked gravel and sand, stones, moss and meticulously pruned trees is in Kyoto, particularly at the temples of Ryōan-ji, Kennin-ji and Daitoku-ji. You can sign up for guided meditation sessions at Shunkō-in, a subtemple of Daitoku-ji.

India

India is home to hundreds of ashrams where spiritual seekers can study and practise meditation across a number of traditions. Buddhism is of strong historical importance here and one of the most sacred sites in India is Bodh Gaya in Bihar, where Buddha achieved enlightenment, and it should be at the top of your list for a meditation pilgrimage. You can also join the throngs of overseas visitors looking for spiritual awakening at McLeod Ganj in Dharamshala where his Holiness the Dalai Lama resides, surrounded by forest and at the edge of the Himalayas. You'll find a number of centres offering meditation courses in the nearby villages of Bhagsu and Dharamkot.

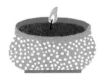

MEDITATION AT HOME

Find a comfortable, quiet spot to sit at home where you won't be interrupted or distracted. If you're a beginner meditator, start with just a few minutes at a time – a short daily practice is more beneficial than a longer practice once a week. Here are a few meditation techniques you can try to see what works for you.

Chanting

Think of a mantra – it can be one word ('Om' is often used) or a phrase that's meaningful to you – and then say it aloud over and over. By doing so, the vibrations will help to calm your mind and the repetition will help you to focus rather than letting your mind wander.

Breath awareness

This technique encourages mindfulness through focusing on your breathing. Close your eyes and focus on your breath, noticing as you breathe in and out. It's okay to let your mind drift to thoughts; just gently acknowledge when it does and then bring your focus back to your breath.

Mandala colouring

Considered sacred symbols, mandalas ('circle' in Sanskrit) are said to represent the universe and are used in meditation for focusing attention and encouraging introspection. In this technique, you mindfully colour-in geometric shapes to promote relaxation and calm. You can buy mandala colouring books or make your own by following instructions online.

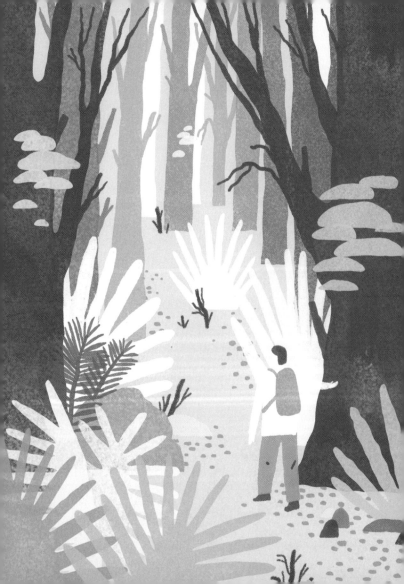

Nature immersion

In our device-dominant world with the never-ending demands of work, home and family commitments, there's a greater need than ever to find ways of reducing stress, ways to reconnect with ourselves and calm the mind and body. This book discusses treating yourself to a day spa, seeking out Ayurveda treatments, going to a creative workshop and spending time at a yoga retreat. But if you're looking for the most simple and affordable method, look no further than your own backyard.

.

Research suggests far too many of us, particularly in the Western world, are not getting enough fresh air or time in our natural surroundings. While just getting outside for an hour a day is a good start, the practice of nature immersion involves connecting to nature on a deeper level. Often when we're outside we're glued to our phones or generally distracted. Truly immersing yourself in your natural surrounds means consciously observing what's around you, what you see, what you hear, what you can touch. By doing this your mind is focused, clear and not thinking about that work presentation or what you need to buy at the shops.

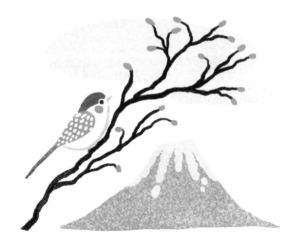

One type of nature immersion is the concept of forest bathing. Also known as shinrin-yoku, forest bathing was developed in Japan in the 1980s. While Japan might be synonymous with giant neon billboards, bullet trains silently whooshing by and a landscape of glittering glass skyscrapers, around two-thirds of the country is actually covered in forest. The high-stress work demands of Japan's economic boom in the 1980s were taking a toll on the nation's health, so shinrin-yoku was devised as a way to self-heal by reconnecting with nature on a deeper level – taking a slow walk, breathing in the fresh air and being hyper-conscious of your external environment.

To experience healing nature immersion, you don't need to drive for hours to find a mountain to climb or head off to the nearest rainforest either. Once you cultivate an awareness of nature, you'll be surprised at what you will find in your local park or even what your own balcony or garden can offer. Listen to the birds, inspect what's going on in the flowerbeds or lawn, keep an eye out for butterflies or insects that flit past you on your balcony. Get all David Attenborough with what you have to work with – nature is all around us all the time.

WHAT'S SO GOOD ABOUT IT?

The reported physical and mental health benefits are extensive and varied. Being in nature reduces stress as we are able to disconnect from our worries, demands and negative thoughts. The more you focus your awareness on what's happening around you in nature, the more in the present you are and the less time you have to worry about anything else.

Studies conducted by Dr Qing Li, author of *Forest Bathing: How Trees Can Help You Find Health and Happiness* and one of the leading experts on forest bathing, from Tokyo's Nippon Medical School, show that spending time in nature increased the body's natural killer cells, the cells that help to fight off cancer. Research also shows that trees emit natural phytoncides, and exposure to these can improve sleep, strengthen the immune system and lower stress hormones.

Spending time in nature can also boost our creativity by giving the mind a chance to slow down and reset. Walking mindfully through a forest or sitting calmly by a beautiful lake will help you avoid burnout and leave you with an improved sense of wellbeing. Intentional nature immersion can also help alleviate anxiety and depression.

THE BEST PLACES FOR NATURE IMMERSION

Beyond your own backyard, you can try reconnecting with nature anywhere in the world, but here are a few countries that revere the natural world.

Canada

With a staggering number of national parks and an eye-popping natural landscape, Canada offers a ridiculous amount of nature immersion opportunities – it's a wonder Canadians are ever found indoors. You can head off into the lush wilderness of Banff National Park, where hiking trails are sometimes shared with grizzlies and faster-than-you-would-ever-expect moose, or explore the endless Arctic landscape keeping an eye out for soft-toy-like-but-terrifying polar bears. The famous runs at Whistler beckon snowboarders while those looking for less action will find plenty of remote sandy beaches to simply wander mindfully along.

New Zealand

Of course the setting used for *The Lord of the Rings* films has to be up there as one of the best countries in which to get back to nature. New Zealand is a land of lush undulating hills, mountains dusted in snow, bays of turquoise waters, golden stretches of empty beaches, otherworldly volcanic landscapes and curtains of water crashing down from epic waterfalls. Nature is not hard to find here and all you need to do is figure out how you'd like to immerse yourself in it. Tackle one of the country's mighty Great Walks, perhaps the glorious Abel Tasman National Park's iconic Coast Track; paddle a kayak on inky waters surrounded by imposing cliffs in Milford Sound and spot dolphins frolicking; or take to the famous ski slopes for some wild back-country action.

Norway

Norway is a land of incredible beauty with glorious fjords, epic icefields and imposing mountain peaks providing the ultimate landscape for nature lovers. And that's exactly what the typical Norwegian is. A love of the wild outdoors and being at one with nature is wrapped up in the Norwegian term friluftsliv (pronounced free-loofts-leev), which can be loosely translated as 'free air life'. Norwegians engage with nature with deep respect and, as a result, reap the benefits, consistently ranking high on the list of the world's happiest countries, partly attributed to a lifestyle that is at one with the natural world. Whether you wish to hike a mountain in Jotunheimen National Park, shoosh down the powdery slopes of any number of the country's ski resorts or see all its wintry wilderness wonder from the back of a dog sled, Norway is the quintessential nature immersion destination.

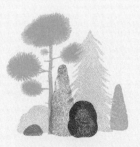

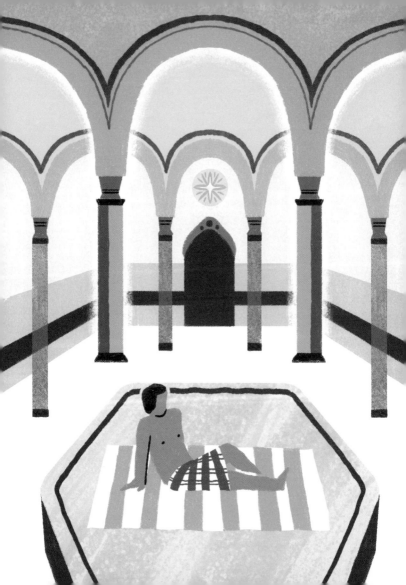

Saunas and bathhouses

The ways in which people socialise, connect, ponder life's big questions and simply spend quality time together differ around the world. Some cultures take to the local pub to knock back a cold one; some gather over bountiful, lengthy feasts in the home; others like to get sweaty together — not in that way — in a sauna or a public bathhouse. Saunas in the West are often found in gyms and used purely for a quick steam post-workout, while the thought of public communal bathing may be enough to give up washing for good. But for other cultures, these places are sacred and not only benefit health and wellbeing but also serve as important communal gathering places, and have done so for centuries. Here are the bathhouse methods of three particular cultures.

.

SAUNA

The Finns came up with the idea of the sauna, which makes sense given that Finland is situated in the extreme north of Europe and right up there as one of the coldest countries on the planet. But the sauna is not just a place to get toasty, it's an important part of Finnish culture. Many people have a sauna in their home and it's considered an honour to be invited to it. Saunas offer a steamy sanctuary where the Finns can purify their minds and bodies, socialise and take a meditative break. It's also where a lot of business dealings are negotiated and important decisions are made.

HAMMAM

In Turkey, the hammam – a traditional public bathhouse – is where people congregate for a steam to sweat out impurities, indulge in a massage (in reality, a decent body bashing) and get a good scrub down, but also to catch up on the latest local gossip. It is part of deep cultural and religious traditions and is associated with Islam's focus on personal cleanliness and ablution rituals. The steam bath originated with the Romans and was introduced to the Byzantines who then passed it onto the Turks who gave it the name hammam. Commonly found throughout the Middle East and North Africa, hammams are generally gender-segregated and often housed in awe-inspiring historical architectural buildings, adding to the experience.

BANYA

Russia, another chilly spot on the world map, is also fond of a little warming up and, to do so, Russians take to their version of a sauna, the banya, which is deeply ingrained in Russian culture. The main feature of a banya is the steam room (parilka), similar to the Finnish sauna, where rocks are heated and water is poured over them to produce steam (often pine oil drops are added to the water for an invigorating aroma). And just to keep things interesting, it's common practice when taking a banya to get a lashing from a stranger with a bunch of twigs (venik) to the point of stinging (said to improve circulation) and then plunge yourself into an icy pool afterwards. Ah, relaxing.

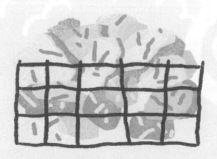

WHAT'S SO GOOD ABOUT IT?

With a temperature of around 80–100°C
(176–212°F), a sauna can have you
sweating like you're in a chilli-eating
comp and breathing like you're Darth
Vader, but the experience can offer a
number of benefits for body and mind.
Sweating up a storm helps the body
to release toxins and impurities and
it can aid in weight loss. The steam
from a sauna, banya or hammam can
improve blood flow, which is good for
circulation and speeds up recovery after
exercise, and it helps skin look better, too.
It's also a great way to relieve stress and
take a break for the mind as well as
the body.

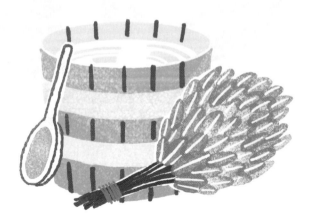

Finland

For the ultimate Finnish sauna experience, visit Jätkänkämppä in the town of Kuopio where the traditional smoke sauna is housed in a cosy, rustic log cabin with smoke-blackened walls – it doesn't get more authentic than this. It's set at the edge of a lake so you can brave a frigid dip at the end of your sauna. If you're after something more modern, try the ultra-hip Löyly located on Helsinki's waterfront. There's a choice of a traditional smoke sauna and a wood-burning sauna, and a smaller one for private bookings.

Turkey

Step inside the simply stunning interior of Istanbul's Kılıç Ali Paşa Hamamı, built in 1580, for a quintessential Turkish hammam experience. The service is five-star and you'll feel like a royal – an extremely clean one – when you leave. The grand Ayasofya Hürrem Sultan Hamamı, built across the road from Aya Sofya (Hagia Sophia) in 1556, underwent a three-year, multimillion-dollar restoration just under a decade ago and offers an impressively luxurious hammam experience in Istanbul's Old City.

Russia

Moscow's spectacular Sanduny Baths is the oldest banya in the city and an essential stop on any visit to Moscow. The interiors are like something from a museum with Baroque, Rococo and Gothic features, intricate woodcarving and an air of historic grandeur. Bathing areas are gender-segregated and private rooms are available. This is the perfect place to rejuvenate after a day of pounding the city streets and is particularly soul-soothing on a freezing winter's day.

Visiting a bathhouse

Generally, if you're visiting a sauna, banya or hammam,
you're doing it sans clothing. Nuding up is de rigueur and
usually places are separated by gender. When it comes to
public hammams, some places will ask men and women
to keep their underwear on, and in many places it's
fine to leave your swimsuit on if you're not comfortable
going au naturel, though that will probably elicit more
staring than if you were starkers.

If you're a first-timer, here are a few guiding
points to remember.

.

FOR A SAUNA

- Shower first before going inside the sauna.

- Sit on your towel.

- Use a ladle to throw water on the sauna stove, which will then give off steam; usually this is done by the person closest to the stove.

- Sometimes a bunch of birch twigs called a vasta or vihta (depending on the region) is used to lightly whip the skin to improve circulation.

- When you've had enough, jump in the lake if there's one handy or hop under a cold shower to refresh.

- A cold beer is considered the crucial final step, of course.

FOR A HAMMAM

- Enter the hammam and pay at the counter – ask for the traditional style where you'll receive an attendant's service.

- Head to the change room, strip off and slip on your flip-flops or sandals.

- Find a spot on the göbektaşı (the raised central platform), pop your mat down and let the steam do its thing.

- After around 15 minutes of steaming, your attendant will give you a good scrub down (gommage) like someone sandpapering your skin off, followed by a short massage, before a final cold rinse to shock you back to life.

FOR A BANYA

- Strip off in the change room before entering the parilka (steam room).

- If felt hats are available, pop one on your head. It might look a little, ah, unfashionable, but it helps protect your hair from the intense heat.

- Relax and enjoy the detoxification process of the steam, but don't overdo it. If you feel light-headed, take a break. Some banya have cold plunge pools for this reason.

- Pick up a venik (a bunch of birch tree branches) and give yourself a light whipping or if someone offers to do it for you kindly accept and then return the favour afterwards.

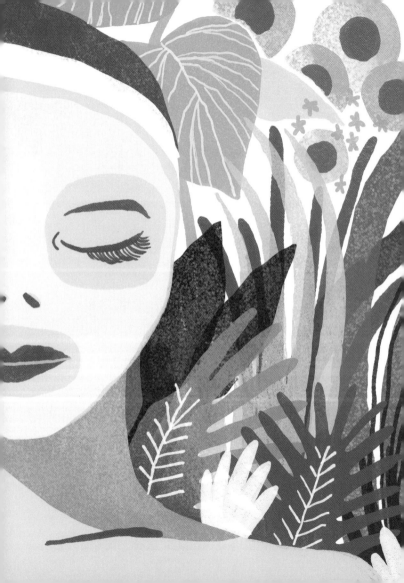

Spa treatments

Dahhling, let's day spa. While day spas were once the domain of high-flying businesspeople, models and celebrities, these days it seems more and more of us are wrapping ourselves in a cloud-like robe, slipping our feet into terry-towelling slippers and indulging in spa treatments to soothe our frazzled minds and knotted-up bodies.

.

Taking time out for a bit of self-love is a crucial step towards mental and physical wellbeing. It's a way of telling yourself you deserve to feel good, of recognising that you do need a break from the demands of daily life and of checking in with your mind and body regularly as a means of self-awareness. Sure, fancy day spas aren't at the heart of finding self-love, but they certainly serve as a delightful way to treat and nurture ourselves in the pursuit of it.

Day spas and spa resorts vary widely in the facilities, price tags and services offered, but you'll generally find a range of massages (*see* p. 47 for more about massage), facials and body treatments on the menu. And in the lotions and potions expect a variety of ingredients, from the standard to the 'Excuse me, what?' with coconut oil, honey, sea salt, mud, rose, seaweed and coffee regularly on the list, occasionally alongside bathing in a barrel of wine, being rubbed in diamond dust, peeling layers of skin off with acid or having snails crawl over your face!

If you can't make it to a day spa, you can turn your home into one instead (*see* p. 78).

FACIALS
Generally, a standard facial will consist of a few basic steps starting with a cleanse and exfoliate followed by a massage, mask and moisturiser. A qualified beautician should analyse your skin beforehand and recommend the most suitable facial for your skin type. Specialised facials for specific skin issues are usually available, too.

BODY TREATMENTS

Most spas offer a number of different body treatments including body scrubs, polishes, wraps and signature treatments. Body scrubs might involve a sugar, salt or coffee-grounds mixture used to exfoliate the skin and remove dead skin cells. Afterwards you hop under the shower for a rinse before your moisturising or detoxifying wrap, where you'll be lucky enough to relax for about 20–30 minutes all warm and wrapped up like a beauty-queen burrito.

VICHY SHOWERS

Many spas also offer Vichy showers, a type of aquatherapy. This typically involves lying on a wooden bed in a wet room under a line of showerheads, which rain down water for a deeply relaxing massage.

Fancy day spas aren't at the heart of finding self-love, but they certainly serve as a delightful way to treat and nurture ourselves.

WHAT'S SO GOOD ABOUT IT?

The question really is what's *not* good about a day spa? These temples to pampering are there to help you indulge, relax and de-stress. Facials, body scrubs and massages all work to get rid of dead skin cells, eliminate toxins, improve circulation, stimulate the lymphatic system, and moisturise and rehydrate the skin to make it look brighter and healthier.

Beyond the physical, day spas give you time for pure rest and relaxation. This activates your parasympathetic nervous system, often called your 'rest and digest' system, and allows your body to recover from the stress and adrenaline rushes you may deal with in your everyday life.

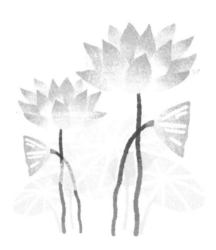

THE BEST SPA EXPERIENCES

The Dolder Spa, Switzerland
Part of the Dolder Grand, a first-class fairytale-like hotel in Zurich, this award-winning spa is centred around a striking indoor black-tiled pool with winding stone walls and stunning views over Lake Zurich. If you can tear yourself away from this scene, the spa has an extensive menu of bespoke treatments including facials, anti-ageing skin treatments and detox scrubs and wraps. The spa's signature Hydraheaven treatment lives up to its name with a foot bath and massage, dry body scrub, mini-facial, massage and time to let it all go in the massaging waterbed.

Chiva-Som, Thailand
A pioneer of health and wellness resorts in Asia, Chiva-Som has been going strong since 1995 and is one of the leading luxury destinations for nourishing the mind and body. The resort is located in Hua Hin by the beach and the number of different services on offer is overwhelming, but expert staff are there to guide you. Try the Mien facial acupressure, where a therapist taps the meridian channels on the face to cleanse the lymphatic vessels and release tension; this practice also relieves headaches and sinus problems. For something more indulgent, the Siam Ritual Cocoon will have you floating out of the treatment room after your body has been scrubbed, oiled and moisturised with cleansing and nourishing ingredients such as sea salt, body butter and aloe vera.

COMO Shambhala Estate, Bali
Just north of Ubud and surrounded by lush tropical forest, COMO Shambhala Estate will have your muscles loosened, your headaches gone and your mood boosted before you've even made it to your spa treatment booking. The retreat blends traditional Balinese architecture with state-of-the-art facilities, and nature provides the soundtrack as you are immersed in any number of the excellent treatments on offer, from reflexology and a detoxifying Dead Sea mud wrap to a Watsu aquatic therapy massage and a traditional Balinese body wrap with warming spices.

Do-it-yourself
day spa

While a day of being scrubbed, rubbed, massaged
and pampered at a sparkling white-decor day spa is
the ultimate self-care luxury, it can also be tough to
find the time, not to mention the funds, with which
to do it. If, for whatever reason, you can't get to an
indulgent day spa at the moment, it doesn't mean you
need to miss out on pampering. Why not bring the day
spa to you? With a little creativity and, well, definitely
some imagination, you can re-create a day spa at
home using items you probably already have hanging
around. If you share your house with friends or family,
try to arrange a time when you can have some peace
and quiet. It's hard to truly relax with a blaring TV,
noisy children and constant disruptions.

•

THINGS YOU'LL NEED

· bath salts

· essential oils

· scented candle

· calming music

· body scrub

· hair-conditioning mask

· body moisturiser

· face cloth and towel

· fluffy robe

· bowl for hot water

· herbal tea

Step 1: Run yourself a hot bath, and add in your choice of salts or essential oil.

Step 2: Turn down your bathroom lights, light a candle and pop on some calming music.

Step 3: Use a body scrub to exfoliate all over from head to toe, then quickly rinse off in the shower.

Step 4: Slide into the bath for a lovely, long soak.

Step 5: Slather on a hair-conditioning mask while you soak in the tub, then rinse off at the end.

Step 6: Hop out of the bath when you've had enough, dry off, gently rub in the body moisturiser and slip on your fluffiest robe or comfiest PJs.

Step 7: Give yourself a quick facial. Use essential oil to infuse a bowl of hot water, place a towel over your head and steam for around ten minutes. Cleanse and moisturise, taking a little more time and care than usual.

Step 8: Make yourself a pot of herbal tea, snuggle up in a cosy armchair, put your feet up and relish the fact that there's no bill to fix up or traffic to sit in on your way home.

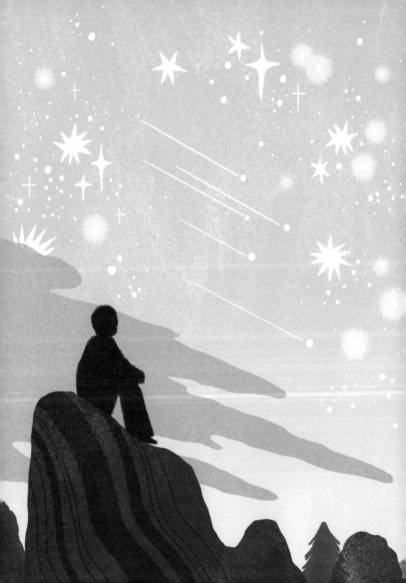

Stargazing

Humans have been looking to the night sky and its dazzling stars in wonderment for millennia. It never ceases to fascinate, humble and spark curiosity. While our ancestors could stare into incredibly dark skies, these days many of us live in urban environments where light pollution is an issue, yet it doesn't stop us from gazing up seeking answers to the mysteries of the world, pondering our place in the magnificence of the universe or simply trying to take a break from the whirl of modern life. Intentional stargazing offers you a chance to slow down, embrace nature and gain perspective on life. Because of this, stargazing as therapy is becoming more and more popular.

Ideally, to get the most out of stargazing, choose a spot away from city lights, smog and pollution. Out in the countryside or wilderness is perfect. Why not take the opportunity for a camping trip at the same time – you can enjoy a break from city life while pondering the stunning celestial bodies glinting high above. But, if getting out to the country is not an option, don't despair – you can look to the sky for therapeutic effects no matter where you are. If you pick a clear night you'll most likely be able to see constellations, planets and the moon on a stargazing session. Who knows, you might even get lucky with a shooting star flashing by for a truly awe-inspiring eyeful. And, if you're keen to become an amateur astronomer, read *Stargazing: Beginners Guide to Astronomy* by Radmila Topalovic and Tom Kerss, published in association with the Royal Observatory Greenwich.

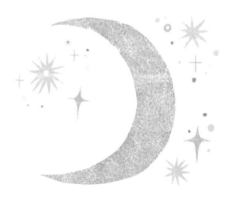

TIPS FOR STARGAZING SUCCESS

Check for clear weather; you need a clear, cloud-free night to see some deep-sky objects, and preferably low humidity, too.

Allow time for your eyes to adapt to the dark; this can take up to 30 minutes. By giving your eyes time to adjust to the darkness, you'll get the most from your stargazing experience.

Know whether the moon will be above the horizon as it can act as a form of light pollution. You want it below the horizon when you're looking at the stars. Find the sunset and moonrise times on a website such as timeanddate.com.

Check out constellation charts online. Start off by looking at stars and star charts; on your next trip, look for planets; on the next, galaxies and nebulae. You'll be learning astronomy and relaxing at the same time.

If you are heading into the country and it's really dark, take a red torch. Red light doesn't affect your eyes as much in terms of adapting to the dark.

Use one of these apps to guide your glittery gazing:

- SkySafari
- NASA
- SkyView
- Star Walk 2.

WHAT'S SO GOOD ABOUT IT?

Stargazing is more than just craning your neck to look up at some stars for a few minutes before heading back inside to watch TV. It's a purposeful, mindful activity that requires patience and concentration. When we lay out a soft blanket, lie on our back and gaze up into the dark expanse, we feel calm and realise that we are connecting to something a whole lot bigger than ourselves. Focusing on constellations, galaxies, planets and the moon helps to put life into perspective – our day-to-day problems, worries and difficulties start to feel, in the scheme of things, often very insignificant.

When you head off on a stargazing session, you are also getting outdoors and into nature, away from phones, TVs and laptops. It allows you to disconnect and slow down, to contemplate and reflect. This benefits mental and physical wellbeing; it reduces anxiety and stress; and it can stimulate creative thinking and productivity.

THE BEST PLACES FOR STARGAZING

Astrotourism is on the rise and people are seeking out dark-sky destinations around the world, often fuelled by a real interest in the night sky as well as the desire to get away from it all, considering some of the best places to stargaze are quite remote. So what is a dark-sky destination? An official dark-sky destination is determined by the International Dark-Sky Association (IDA), which identifies several criteria that need to be met for a site to be designated bronze, silver or gold, depending on the conditions there and what you can see. There are around 130 certified International Dark Sky Places (IDSPs) around the world; here are some of the best picks.

NamibRand Nature Reserve, Namibia

NamibRand Nature Reserve was the first reserve in Africa to be accredited as a dark-sky destination by IDA in 2012 and it has been awarded gold status. The extremely dry weather and clear skies here in the Namib Desert are perfect conditions for staring at the heavens.

Elqui Valley, Chile

In the Atacama Desert, this remote location is another bright star on the growing list of astrotourism hotspots. Given the Elqui Valley's high elevation and cloud-free sky, which is lit up at night with swirls of vivid blue and deep plum, it's no surprise that in 2015 it was declared by IDA as the world's first Dark Sky Sanctuary. It's officially named the Gabriela Mistral Dark Sky Sanctuary after a Chilean poet.

Western Australian outback, Australia

If you're looking for dark skies, they don't come much more inky than the vast Western Australian outback. It's the perfect canvas for taking in the splendour of the mighty Milky Way stretched across the sky, and a number of national parks in the state make ideal stargazing bases.

Mauna Kea, Hawaii

Home to one of the largest telescopes in the world, Hawaii's dormant Mauna Kea volcano on the Big Island is a classic pilgrimage spot for dark-sky enthusiasts. Begin by viewing the epic sunset from the summit observatories (take note, at an altitude of 4205 metres (13,796 feet), altitude sickness is a real risk) and, when these close at nightfall, drive down to the visitor centre from where you can observe the starry show through the visitor telescopes.

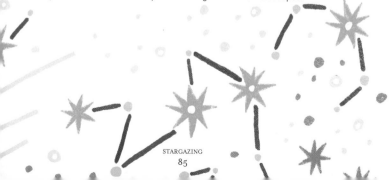

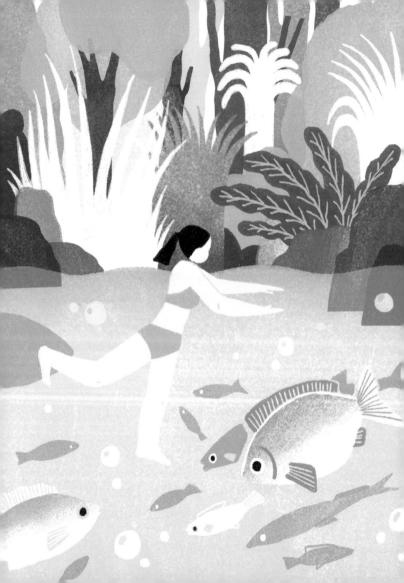

Wild swimming

Swimming is an excellent form of exercise: it works the entire body, builds muscle tone and strength, is easy on the joints and is great for cardiovascular fitness. When done indoors, it is often accompanied by the stink of chlorine, the high-pitched squeal of children splashing about and the annoyance of bumping elbows with other swimmers in busy lap lanes. Swimming isn't just about the physical benefits — it can be therapeutic and hugely beneficial for mental health, too — but it's difficult to reap the rewards with all those distractions around. That's where wild swimming comes in — simply taking swimming back outdoors into nature.

For centuries, people have been taking icy plunges, enjoying relaxing dips or swimming laps in rivers, oceans, ponds and lagoons. There is now a resurgence of interest in wild swimming; its popularity is increasing as people strive to escape from the noise of modern life. Those living in high-density cities are often more than ever disconnected from nature and open-air swimming provides a way of reconnecting with the wild world. When you sink into the water, reeds tickling at your ankles or sand under your feet, sun peeking through the clouds and glinting off the water's surface, trees swaying above you in the breeze, and feel that sense of calm and peace slide over your body, you'll understand why.

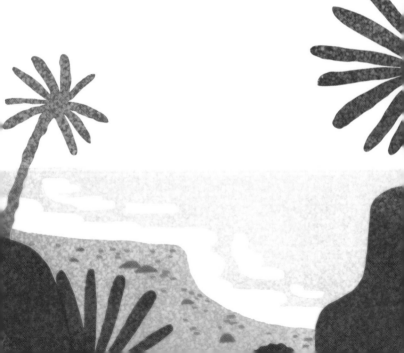

WHAT'S SO GOOD ABOUT IT?

Swapping the chemical-filled water and poor air quality of an indoor pool for fresh air and an open body of water surrounded by forest, bush and emerald hills or bordered by a long stretch of golden sand offers many health benefits. First, just being out in Mother Nature is nourishing for the soul, mind and body, providing clarity, calmness and a chance to switch off. Second, by focusing on your swimming, you are in the present moment and it becomes a meditative activity. Breath technique is an important part of swimming and this attention to breath also puts us in a state of mindfulness, similar to the way a yoga or meditation session does. It slows down the mind so that other thoughts and worries can't linger. This can help with symptoms of anxiety and depression.

Specifically cold-water immersion or winter swimming is a mental and physical endeavour that requires strength and resilience. Plunging into frigid waters for a swim is a way of challenging yourself and the more you do it the more resilience you build up. This character trait can help you deal with any issues or emotional trauma you might be facing out of the water. While evidence-based research is limited, anecdotal evidence suggests that cold-water swimming can reduce chronic pain, improve sleep and boost dopamine levels (the happy hormone) for improved mood.

> There's a resurgence of interest in wild swimming as people strive to escape from the noise of modern life.

SAFE SWIMMING

Wild swimming is not without risks, so keep these things in mind before you start.

There's safety in numbers. Don't go it alone, it's safer to swim with at least one other person in case you find yourself in trouble.

Don't dive into unknown waters. If you don't know the depth of the water, test it first or simply don't dive or jump in so as to avoid injury. Ease into the water instead.

Be aware of any currents or rip tides. Know how to identify these and how to safely swim out of them.

Ice-cold water presents its own risks including cold shock, hypothermia and cardiac arrest. Seek medical advice first if you have a heart condition, asthma or high blood pressure, or are pregnant.

THE BEST PLACES FOR WILD SWIMMING

Hampstead Heath Ponds, England

These cherished institutions in the woods of London's Hampstead Heath are a tranquil respite from the hectic city streets. Dug as reservoirs in the 17th and 18th centuries, the ponds have been attracting swimmers since the early 20th century. People take to these murky brown waters (despite appearances, water quality is high) for pleasure, exercise, therapy and a cool-off when the elusive London sun decides to warm things up. There are three ponds: the Kenwood Ladies' Pond, the Highgate Men's Bathing Pond and the Mixed Pond.

Cenote X'Kekén y Samulá, Mexico

On a scorching summer day in Mexico's Yucatán Peninsula, there is nothing quite like the experience of paddling around in a cenote – a deep, natural swimming hole formed when limestone bedrock collapses revealing a surreal underground pool. Originating from the Mayan word meaning 'well', cenotes were the main water source for the Mayans who considered them to be sacred places and a passage to the underworld. The Yucatán is scattered with awe-inspiring cenotes but one of the most impressive and ideal for swimming is Cenote X'Kekén y Samulá. Sunlight streams in from the top, the water is glass-clear allowing you to see the fish flitting by and long tree roots drape from the ceiling.

Gunlom Plunge Pool, Australia

Australia's World Heritage–listed Kakadu National Park in the Northern Territory is home to the magical Gunlom Plunge Pool. A steep, sweaty walk from the carpark is required to reach the top, but the reward is a large emerald-green waterhole that's fed by a seasonal waterfall, nestled atop a rocky outcrop with expansive views of Kakadu. While it mightn't be the perfect place to rack up your laps, it's an exquisite spot to simply soak in the dramatic scenery of the Australian bush and let your thoughts wander off.

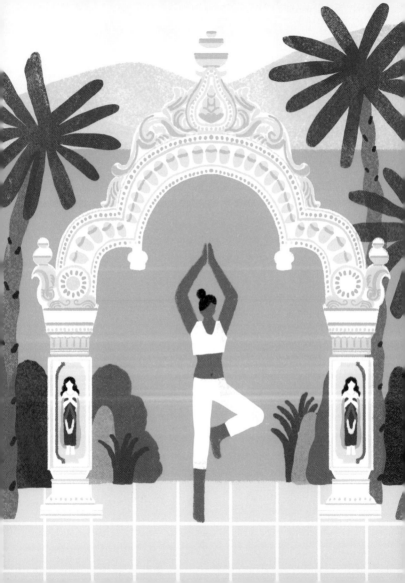

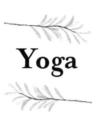

Yoga

Throw on your comfiest workout clothes as it's time
to get on the mat for some yoga. If you've ever played
the game Twister, then you're more than ready to bust
out some of yoga's classic moves such as downward-
facing dog, corpse pose, warrior II and cat-cow,
to list just a few.

·

A practice for the mind and body, yoga is rooted in ancient Indian philosophy and is thought to date as far back as 5000 years ago. Yoga involves a combination of physical postures (asana), breathing techniques (pranayama) and meditation (dhyana). There are a number of yoga styles out there and it's worth trying out different ones to find what suits you best. Are you all about the headstand and using props to stretch and contort your body into shapes? Or do you feel more aligned with a restorative, gentle yoga flow focusing on holding poses longer and deep breathing instead of working up a sweat?

Some of the more popular yoga styles include hatha (a traditional simple style using poses), ashtanga (another traditional style that follows a sequence of poses), Iyengar (a style that focuses on alignment and uses props in poses), vinyasa (a more vigorous, fast-paced fluid style) and Bikram (a sequence of 26 poses practised in a hot room, usually around 40°C (104°F), and good for those who don't mind working out to an aroma of body odour).

WHAT'S SO GOOD ABOUT IT?

The reported list of health benefits of yoga is long and varied, which is why yoga keeps growing more and more popular around the world. Research suggests it increases flexibility and muscle tone, aids in weight loss and improves cardiovascular fitness. By focusing on the breath and being in the moment, yoga relaxes the mind and body, which reduces stress and can help relieve anxiety and depression. Certain poses can have specific benefits, such as assisting the digestive system and helping to reduce period pain.

THE BEST PLACES FOR YOGA

Mysuru (Mysore), India
India is the home of yoga so of course there are hundreds of schools and ashrams all over the country, but you need to do your homework – for every highly acclaimed ashram there are dozens of substandard ones out there, so choose wisely.

The beguiling city of Mysuru (Mysore) in India's south is a magnet for yoga fanatics from all over the world, this being the home of ashtanga and its own Mysore Style established by K Pattabhi Jois. Yoga is taken seriously here and most visitors commit to at least a one-month stay to perfect the art as much as possible. Two of the most well regarded yoga centres are Kpjay Shala and Indea Yoga.

Rishikesh, India
The spiritual town of Rishikesh, set on the banks of the River Ganges in the foothills of the Himalayas, is known for three things: Transcendental Meditation, yoga and the Beatles (the band stayed at an ashram here in 1968 and wrote many of the songs that ended up on their *White Album*). While you're not going to get to see the Beatles, the town is considered the birthplace of yoga so it's the perfect place for a yoga pilgrimage. Yoga centres and ashrams are ubiquitous in Rishikesh and you can practise this ancient art at some of the country's most respected places, including Parmarth Niketan, Phool Chatti and Omkarananda Ganga Sadan.

Bali, Indonesia
The beautiful island of Bali has two sides: on one hand it attracts partygoers looking to let loose in the frenetic nightlife of Kuta and Legian and, on the other, the paradisiacal backdrops, rich culture and spiritual serenity of the island tempt those looking to find themselves, lose themselves, restore and rejuvenate. Ubud, in particular, is a prime spot for getting in touch with your inner yogi – its petal-strewn streets, rice paddies and languid pace lull you into relaxation before you've even rolled out your mat. One of the most popular yoga centres here is the Yoga Barn, which offers a range of classes in different yoga styles.

Yoga at home

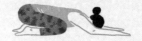

The beauty of yoga is that if you can't hop on a plane to India or Bali at the moment, or you don't like the idea of contorting yourself in front of a class of strangers, it's easy enough to practise from the comfort of your own home. Yoga mats are inexpensive and there are thousands of yoga videos floating around the internet to guide you.

•

Here are a few tips and poses for your home practice:

· Wear loose, comfortable clothing.

· Remember to breathe. Paying attention to your breath is one of the most important aspects of practising yoga.

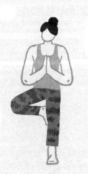

· It's best not to eat a full meal for at least 90 minutes before your practice.

· A regular practice, even if short, will have more benefits than an occasional long practice.

Downward-facing dog (Adho mukha svanasana)

1. Start on all fours (hands and knees) with hands slightly forward of shoulders, knees in line with hips.

2. Press palms into the mat and curl toes under.

3. Breathe in and on the exhale lift knees off the ground, bringing your body into an inverted V, with knees slightly bent and feet hip-width apart.

4. Hold for 30 seconds to one minute.

Child's pose (Balasana)

1. Sit on your heels and move knees so they are hip-width apart.

2. Breathe in and on the exhale move your torso to lay between your thighs, resting your head in front of you on the mat.

3. Place hands on the floor behind you with palms facing up.

4. This is a restful pose and can be used when you need to take a break, so relax your whole body and hold for at least 30 seconds and up to a few minutes.

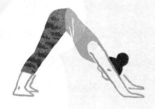

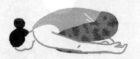

Warrior II (Virabhadrasana II)

1. Stand with legs apart and reach arms out to the sides with palms facing down.

2. Turn right foot 90 degrees to the right and align left heel with right heel.

3. Bend right knee so it's over the ankle, no further. Press left heel firmly into the mat and tuck tailbone in.

4. Turn your head to look to the right and hold pose for 30 seconds to one minute. Repeat on the other side.

Cobra pose (Bhujangasana)

1. Lie face down on the floor and place your hands palms down underneath or next to the shoulders.

2. Press your thighs, pubic bone and tops of your feet into the mat.

3. On an exhale, slowly straighten your arms, keeping the elbows close to your body and slightly bent (or a lot bent if you're doing a modified version), and lift your chest off the mat.

4. Draw your shoulders down the back of your body and gently push the chest forward. Keep the pubic bone pressing down.

5. Hold for 30 seconds.

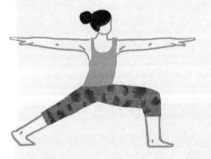

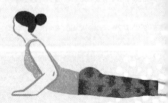

Cat-cow (Marjariasana-bitilasana)

1. Position yourself on all fours with wrists in line with shoulders and knees in line with hips. Look down and slightly in front of you.

2. Inhale and drop your belly, lift your chin and chest towards the ceiling.

3. Exhale and draw your belly towards your spine, releasing your head towards the floor and curving your spine towards the ceiling like a cat stretching.

4. Repeat 5–10 times in a gentle flow.

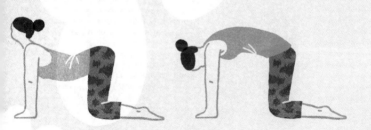

Acknowledgements

I'd like to say a huge thanks to Melissa Kayser, Megan Cuthbert and all the team at Hardie Grant Travel who worked on making this book happen and for the opportunity. A big thank you to my editor, Alexandra Payne, for her excellent suggestions and for really whipping this book into shape. And thanks to Wenjia Tang for her beautiful illustrations. Thanks also to everyone who offered their expertise and assistance in my research for this book, particularly Sandra Jelly from Pink Spirit Yoga, Rev. Takafumi Kawakami from Shunko-in, Dr Qing Li at the Nippon Medical School and Bharath Shetty from Indea Yoga. And, finally, thank you to my husband, Trent, for your endless encouragement, ideas, support and laughs.

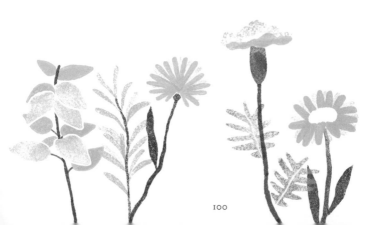

About the author

Kate Morgan is a freelance writer and editor who has worked on a number of guidebooks for Lonely Planet, as well as having written numerous feature stories for clients such as BBC Travel and Condé Nast Traveller. Her job has taken her on plenty of adventures across the globe over the years, including to Japan, Zimbabwe, Amsterdam, Russia, Phuket, India and around Australia. At times, Kate has had the gruelling task of receiving indulgent massages in luxury day spas, participated in Buddhist meditation in Japan, worked out the kinks in yoga sessions in India and sweated out the toxins in a Russian banya, all in the name of research. Kate was also the commissioning editor and contributor to Lonely Planet's *Wellness Escapes* book.

About the illustrator

Wenjia Tang is a freelance illustrator who graduated from Maryland Institute College of Art in 2017. She was born in south-east China, and went to the United States for high school when she was 15. She loves all kinds of animals, and lives with a cat in Manhattan, New York.

Her work has been recognised by American Illustration, Society of Illustrators, *Communication Arts*, AOI, *3x3 Magazine* and more.

Published in 2021 by Hardie Grant Travel,
a division of Hardie Grant Publishing

Hardie Grant Travel (Melbourne)
Building 1, 658 Church Street
Richmond, Victoria 3121

Hardie Grant Travel (Sydney)
Level 7, 45 Jones Street
Ultimo, NSW 2007

www.hardiegrant.com/au/travel

A catalogue record for this
book is available from the
National Library of Australia

NATIONAL
LIBRARY
OF AUSTRALIA

Hardie Grant acknowledges the Traditional Owners of the country
on which we work, the Wurundjeri people of the Kulin nation and the
Gadigal people of the Eora nation, and recognises their continuing
connection to the land, waters and culture. We pay our respects to
their Elders past, present and emerging.

Destination Wellness
ISBN 9781741176896

10 9 8 7 6 5 4 3 2 1

Publisher
Melissa Kayser

Senior editor
Megan Cuthbert

Design
Michelle Mackintosh

Project editor
Alexandra Payne

Proofreader
Rosanna Dutson

Typesetting
Megan Ellis

Colour reproduction by Megan Ellis and Splitting Image Colour Studio
Printed and bound in China by LEO Paper Products LTD.